THIS BOOK BELONGS TO

_____

Date _____

How are you feeling today? _____

I have eaten...

BREAKFAST	WHAT TIME?	Calories

LUNCH	WHAT TIME?	Calories

DINNER	WHAT TIME?	Calories

SNACKS	WHAT TIME?	Calories

TOTAL CALORIES _____

I have exercised...

DOING?	TIME	Calories Burned

TOTAL CALORIES BURNED _____

I have slept...

_____ HOURS

I have drank...

_____ CUPS OF WATER

Meds/vitamins taken

_____

_____

_____

FINAL CALORIES _____
(Calories eaten - calories burned)

Weight today? _____

Change? +/- _____

Date

How are you feeling today?

I have eaten... | I have exercised...

BREAKFAST	WHAT TIME?	Calories	DOING?	TIME	Calories Burned

LUNCH	WHAT TIME?	Calories

TOTAL CALORIES BURNED

I have slept...

HOURS

DINNER	WHAT TIME?	Calories

I have drank...

CUPS OF WATER

Meds/vitamins taken

SNACKS	WHAT TIME?	Calories

TOTAL CALORIES

FINAL CALORIES
(Calories eaten - calories burned)

Weight today?   Change? +/-

Date _____

How are you feeling today? _____

I have eaten...

BREAKFAST	WHAT TIME?	Calories

LUNCH	WHAT TIME?	Calories

DINNER	WHAT TIME?	Calories

SNACKS	WHAT TIME?	Calories

TOTAL CALORIES _____

I have exercised...

DOING?	TIME	Calories Burned

TOTAL CALORIES BURNED _____

I have slept...

_____ HOURS

I have drank...

_____ CUPS OF WATER

Meds/vitamins taken

_____

_____

_____

FINAL CALORIES _____
(Calories eaten - calories burned)

Weight today? _____   **Change? +/-** _____

Date _____

How are you feeling today? _____

I have eaten...

BREAKFAST	WHAT TIME?	Calories

LUNCH	WHAT TIME?	Calories

DINNER	WHAT TIME?	Calories

SNACKS	WHAT TIME?	Calories

TOTAL CALORIES _____

I have exercised...

DOING?	TIME	Calories Burned

TOTAL CALORIES BURNED _____

I have slept...

_____ HOURS

I have drank...

_____ CUPS OF WATER

Meds/vitamins taken

FINAL CALORIES _____
(Calories eaten - calories burned)

Weight today? _____ # Change? +/- _____

Date _____

How are you feeling today? _____

I have eaten...

BREAKFAST	WHAT TIME?	Calories
LUNCH	WHAT TIME?	Calories
DINNER	WHAT TIME?	Calories
SNACKS	WHAT TIME?	Calories
TOTAL CALORIES		

I have exercised...

DOING?	TIME	Calories Burned

TOTAL CALORIES BURNED _____

I have slept...

_____ HOURS

I have drank...

_____ CUPS OF WATER

Meds/vitamins taken

FINAL CALORIES
(Calories eaten - calories burned)

Weight today? _____

Change? +/- _____

Date

How are you feeling today?

I have eaten...

BREAKFAST	WHAT TIME?	Calories
LUNCH	WHAT TIME?	Calories
DINNER	WHAT TIME?	Calories
SNACKS	WHAT TIME?	Calories

TOTAL CALORIES

Weight today?

I have exercised...

DOING?	TIME	Calories Burned

TOTAL CALORIES BURNED

I have slept...

HOURS

I have drank...

CUPS OF WATER

Meds/vitamins taken

FINAL CALORIES
(Calories eaten - calories burned)

Change? +/-

Date _____

How are you feeling today? _____

I have eaten...

BREAKFAST	WHAT TIME?	Calories

LUNCH	WHAT TIME?	Calories

DINNER	WHAT TIME?	Calories

SNACKS	WHAT TIME?	Calories

TOTAL CALORIES _____

I have exercised...

DOING?	TIME	Calories Burned

TOTAL CALORIES BURNED _____

I have slept...

_____ HOURS

I have drank...

_____ CUPS OF WATER

Meds/vitamins taken

_____
_____
_____

FINAL CALORIES _____
(Calories eaten - calories burned)

Weight today? _____   **Change? +/-** _____

Date

How are you feeling today?

I have eaten...

BREAKFAST	WHAT TIME?	Calories
LUNCH	WHAT TIME?	Calories
DINNER	WHAT TIME?	Calories
SNACKS	WHAT TIME?	Calories

TOTAL CALORIES

Weight today?

I have exercised...

DOING?	TIME	Calories Burned

TOTAL CALORIES BURNED

I have slept...

HOURS

I have drank...

CUPS OF WATER

Meds/vitamins taken

FINAL CALORIES
(Calories eaten - calories burned)

Change? +/-

Date _____

How are you feeling today? _____

I have eaten...

BREAKFAST	WHAT TIME?	Calories

LUNCH	WHAT TIME?	Calories

DINNER	WHAT TIME?	Calories

SNACKS	WHAT TIME?	Calories

TOTAL CALORIES _____

I have exercised...

DOING?	TIME	Calories Burned

TOTAL CALORIES BURNED _____

I have slept...

_____ HOURS

I have drank...

_____ CUPS OF WATER

Meds/vitamins taken

_____

_____

_____

FINAL CALORIES _____
(Calories eaten - calories burned)

Weight today? _____

Change? +/- _____

Date _____

How are you feeling today? _____

I have eaten...			I have exercised...		
BREAKFAST	WHAT TIME?	Calories	DOING?	TIME	Calories Burned
LUNCH	WHAT TIME?	Calories			

TOTAL CALORIES BURNED _____

I have slept...

HOURS

DINNER	WHAT TIME?	Calories

I have drank...

CUPS OF WATER

Meds/vitamins taken

SNACKS	WHAT TIME?	Calories

TOTAL CALORIES _____

FINAL CALORIES _____
(Calories eaten - calories burned)

Weight today? _____

Change? +/- _____

Date _____

How are you feeling today? _____

I have eaten...

BREAKFAST	WHAT TIME?	Calories

LUNCH	WHAT TIME?	Calories

DINNER	WHAT TIME?	Calories

SNACKS	WHAT TIME?	Calories

TOTAL CALORIES _____

I have exercised...

DOING?	TIME	Calories Burned

TOTAL CALORIES BURNED _____

I have slept...

_____ HOURS

I have drank...

CUPS OF WATER

Meds/vitamins taken

FINAL CALORIES _____
(Calories eaten - calories burned)

Weight today? _____ Change? +/- _____

Date _____

How are you feeling today? _____

I have eaten...

BREAKFAST	WHAT TIME?	Calories

LUNCH	WHAT TIME?	Calories

DINNER	WHAT TIME?	Calories

SNACKS	WHAT TIME?	Calories

TOTAL CALORIES _____

Weight today? _____

I have exercised...

DOING?	TIME	Calories Burned

TOTAL CALORIES BURNED _____

I have slept...

_____ HOURS

I have drank...

_____ CUPS OF WATER

Meds/vitamins taken

_____
_____
_____

FINAL CALORIES _____
(Calories eaten - calories burned)

Change? +/- _____

Date _____

How are you feeling today? _____

I have eaten...

BREAKFAST	WHAT TIME?	Calories

LUNCH	WHAT TIME?	Calories

DINNER	WHAT TIME?	Calories

SNACKS	WHAT TIME?	Calories

TOTAL CALORIES _____

Weight today? _____

I have exercised...

DOING?	TIME	Calories Burned

TOTAL CALORIES BURNED _____

I have slept...

_____ HOURS

I have drank...

_____ CUPS OF WATER

Meds/vitamins taken

FINAL CALORIES _____
(Calories eaten - calories burned)

Change? +/- _____

Date _____

How are you feeling today? _____

I have eaten...

BREAKFAST	WHAT TIME?	Calories

LUNCH	WHAT TIME?	Calories

DINNER	WHAT TIME?	Calories

SNACKS	WHAT TIME?	Calories

TOTAL CALORIES _____

I have exercised...

DOING?	TIME	Calories Burned

TOTAL CALORIES BURNED _____

I have slept...

_____ HOURS

I have drank...

_____ CUPS OF WATER

Meds/vitamins taken

_____

_____

_____

FINAL CALORIES _____
(Calories eaten - calories burned)

Weight today? _____

Change? +/- _____

Date _____

How are you feeling today? _____

I have eaten...

BREAKFAST	WHAT TIME?	Calories

LUNCH	WHAT TIME?	Calories

DINNER	WHAT TIME?	Calories

SNACKS	WHAT TIME?	Calories

TOTAL CALORIES _____

Weight today? _____

I have exercised...

DOING?	TIME	Calories Burned

TOTAL CALORIES BURNED _____

I have slept...

HOURS _____

I have drank...

CUPS OF WATER _____

Meds/vitamins taken

_____
_____
_____

FINAL CALORIES _____
(Calories eaten - calories burned)

Change? +/- _____

Date _____

How are you feeling today? _____

I have eaten...

BREAKFAST	WHAT TIME?	Calories

LUNCH	WHAT TIME?	Calories

DINNER	WHAT TIME?	Calories

SNACKS	WHAT TIME?	Calories

TOTAL CALORIES _____

I have exercised...

DOING?	TIME	Calories Burned

TOTAL CALORIES BURNED _____

I have slept...

_____ HOURS

I have drank...

CUPS OF WATER

Meds/vitamins taken

_____
_____
_____

FINAL CALORIES _____
(Calories eaten - calories burned)

Weight today? _____

Change? +/- _____

Date _____

How are you feeling today? _____

I have eaten...

BREAKFAST	WHAT TIME?	Calories

LUNCH	WHAT TIME?	Calories

DINNER	WHAT TIME?	Calories

SNACKS	WHAT TIME?	Calories

TOTAL CALORIES _____

I have exercised...

DOING?	TIME	Calories Burned

TOTAL CALORIES BURNED _____

I have slept...

_____ HOURS

I have drank...

_____ CUPS OF WATER

Meds/vitamins taken

_____

_____

_____

FINAL CALORIES _____
(Calories eaten - calories burned)

Weight today? _____

Change? +/- _____

Date _____

How are you feeling today? _____

I have eaten...

BREAKFAST	WHAT TIME?	Calories

LUNCH	WHAT TIME?	Calories

DINNER	WHAT TIME?	Calories

SNACKS	WHAT TIME?	Calories

TOTAL CALORIES _____

Weight today? _____

I have exercised...

DOING?	TIME	Calories Burned

TOTAL CALORIES BURNED _____

I have slept...

HOURS _____

I have drank...

CUPS OF WATER _____

Meds/vitamins taken

_____

_____

_____

FINAL CALORIES _____
(Calories eaten - calories burned)

Change? +/- _____

Date

How are you feeling today?

I have eaten...

BREAKFAST	WHAT TIME?	Calories

LUNCH	WHAT TIME?	Calories

DINNER	WHAT TIME?	Calories

SNACKS	WHAT TIME?	Calories

TOTAL CALORIES

Weight today?

I have exercised...

DOING?	TIME	Calories Burned

TOTAL CALORIES BURNED

I have slept...

HOURS

I have drank...

CUPS OF WATER

Meds/vitamins taken

FINAL CALORIES
(Calories eaten - calories burned)

Change? +/-

Date _____

How are you feeling today? _____

I have eaten...

BREAKFAST	WHAT TIME?	Calories
LUNCH	WHAT TIME?	Calories
DINNER	WHAT TIME?	Calories
SNACKS	WHAT TIME?	Calories
TOTAL CALORIES		

I have exercised...

DOING?	TIME	Calories Burned

TOTAL CALORIES BURNED _____

I have slept...

HOURS

I have drank...

CUPS OF WATER

Meds/vitamins taken

FINAL CALORIES
(Calories eaten - calories burned)

Weight today? _____   # Change? +/- _____

Date _____

How are you feeling today? _____

I have eaten...   # I have exercised...

BREAKFAST	WHAT TIME?	Calories

DOING?	TIME	Calories Burned

LUNCH	WHAT TIME?	Calories

TOTAL CALORIES BURNED _____

I have slept...

_____ HOURS

DINNER	WHAT TIME?	Calories

I have drank...

_____ CUPS OF WATER

Meds/vitamins taken

SNACKS	WHAT TIME?	Calories

TOTAL CALORIES _____

FINAL CALORIES _____
(Calories eaten - calories burned)

Weight today? _____   # Change? +/- _____

Date _____

How are you feeling today? _____

I have eaten...

BREAKFAST	WHAT TIME?	Calories

LUNCH	WHAT TIME?	Calories

DINNER	WHAT TIME?	Calories

SNACKS	WHAT TIME?	Calories

TOTAL CALORIES _____

I have exercised...

DOING?	TIME	Calories Burned

TOTAL CALORIES BURNED _____

I have slept...

_____ HOURS

I have drank...

_____ CUPS OF WATER

Meds/vitamins taken

FINAL CALORIES _____
(Calories eaten - calories burned)

Weight today? _____

Change? +/- _____

Date _____

How are you feeling today? _____

I have eaten...

BREAKFAST	WHAT TIME?	Calories

LUNCH	WHAT TIME?	Calories

DINNER	WHAT TIME?	Calories

SNACKS	WHAT TIME?	Calories

TOTAL CALORIES _____

Weight today? _____

I have exercised...

DOING?	TIME	Calories Burned

TOTAL CALORIES BURNED _____

I have slept...

_____ HOURS

I have drank...

_____ CUPS OF WATER

Meds/vitamins taken

_____

_____

_____

FINAL CALORIES _____
(Calories eaten - calories burned)

Change? +/- _____

Date _____

How are you feeling today? _____

I have eaten...

BREAKFAST	WHAT TIME?	Calories

LUNCH	WHAT TIME?	Calories

DINNER	WHAT TIME?	Calories

SNACKS	WHAT TIME?	Calories

TOTAL CALORIES _____

I have exercised...

DOING?	TIME	Calories Burned

TOTAL CALORIES BURNED _____

I have slept...

HOURS _____

I have drank...

CUPS OF WATER _____

Meds/vitamins taken

FINAL CALORIES _____
(Calories eaten - calories burned)

Weight today? _____

Change? +/- _____

Date _____

How are you feeling today? _____

I have eaten...				I have exercised...		
BREAKFAST	WHAT TIME?	Calories		DOING?	TIME	Calories Burned
LUNCH	WHAT TIME?	Calories				
				TOTAL CALORIES BURNED _____		

I have slept...
_____ HOURS

I have drank...
CUPS OF WATER

Meds/vitamins taken

DINNER	WHAT TIME?	Calories

SNACKS	WHAT TIME?	Calories

TOTAL CALORIES _____

FINAL CALORIES _____
(Calories eaten - calories burned)

Weight today? _____   Change? +/- _____

Date _____ _____

How are you feeling today? _____

I have eaten...

BREAKFAST	WHAT TIME?	Calories

LUNCH	WHAT TIME?	Calories

DINNER	WHAT TIME?	Calories

SNACKS	WHAT TIME?	Calories

TOTAL CALORIES _____

Weight today? _____

I have exercised...

DOING?	TIME	Calories Burned

TOTAL CALORIES BURNED _____

I have slept...

_____ HOURS

I have drank...

_____ CUPS OF WATER

Meds/vitamins taken

_____
_____
_____
_____

FINAL CALORIES _____
(Calories eaten - calories burned)

Change? +/- _____

Date _____

How are you feeling today? _____

I have eaten...

BREAKFAST	WHAT TIME?	Calories

LUNCH	WHAT TIME?	Calories

DINNER	WHAT TIME?	Calories

SNACKS	WHAT TIME?	Calories

TOTAL CALORIES _____

I have exercised...

DOING?	TIME	Calories Burned

TOTAL CALORIES BURNED _____

I have slept...

_____ HOURS

I have drank...

CUPS OF WATER

Meds/vitamins taken

FINAL CALORIES _____
(Calories eaten - calories burned)

Weight today? _____

Change? +/- _____

Date _____

How are you feeling today? _____

I have eaten...

BREAKFAST	WHAT TIME?	Calories

LUNCH	WHAT TIME?	Calories

DINNER	WHAT TIME?	Calories

SNACKS	WHAT TIME?	Calories

TOTAL CALORIES _____

Weight today? _____

I have exercised...

DOING?	TIME	Calories Burned

TOTAL CALORIES BURNED _____

I have slept...

_____ HOURS

I have drank...

_____ CUPS OF WATER

Meds/vitamins taken

_____
_____
_____

FINAL CALORIES _____
(Calories eaten - calories burned)

Change? +/- _____

Date _____

How are you feeling today? _____

I have eaten...

BREAKFAST	WHAT TIME?	Calories

LUNCH	WHAT TIME?	Calories

DINNER	WHAT TIME?	Calories

SNACKS	WHAT TIME?	Calories

TOTAL CALORIES _____

I have exercised...

DOING?	TIME	Calories Burned

TOTAL CALORIES BURNED _____

I have slept...

_____ HOURS

I have drank...

_____ CUPS OF WATER

Meds/vitamins taken

_____
_____
_____
_____

FINAL CALORIES _____
(Calories eaten - calories burned)

Weight today? _____   **Change? +/-** _____

Date

How are you feeling today?

I have eaten...

BREAKFAST	**WHAT TIME?**	Calories
LUNCH	**WHAT TIME?**	Calories
DINNER	**WHAT TIME?**	Calories
SNACKS	**WHAT TIME?**	Calories

TOTAL CALORIES _____

I have exercised...

DOING?	**TIME**	Calories Burned

TOTAL CALORIES BURNED _____

I have slept...

_____ HOURS

I have drank...

_____ CUPS OF WATER

Meds/vitamins taken

FINAL CALORIES _____
(Calories eaten - calories burned)

Weight today? _____

Change? +/- _____

Date _____

How are you feeling today? _____

I have eaten...

BREAKFAST	WHAT TIME?	Calories

LUNCH	WHAT TIME?	Calories

DINNER	WHAT TIME?	Calories

SNACKS	WHAT TIME?	Calories

TOTAL CALORIES _____

I have exercised...

DOING?	TIME	Calories Burned

TOTAL CALORIES BURNED _____

I have slept...

_____ HOURS

I have drank...

_____ CUPS OF WATER

Meds/vitamins taken

_____

_____

_____

_____

FINAL CALORIES _____
(Calories eaten - calories burned)

Weight today? _____   **Change? +/-** _____

Date

How are you feeling today?

I have eaten...

BREAKFAST	WHAT TIME?	Calories
LUNCH	WHAT TIME?	Calories
DINNER	WHAT TIME?	Calories
SNACKS	WHAT TIME?	Calories

TOTAL CALORIES

I have exercised...

DOING?	TIME	Calories Burned

**TOTAL CALORIES
BURNED**

I have slept...

HOURS

I have drank...

CUPS OF
WATER

Meds/vitamins taken

FINAL CALORIES
(Calories eaten - calories burned)

Weight today?

Change? +/-

Date _____

How are you feeling today? _____

I have eaten...

BREAKFAST	WHAT TIME?	Calories

LUNCH	WHAT TIME?	Calories

DINNER	WHAT TIME?	Calories

SNACKS	WHAT TIME?	Calories

TOTAL CALORIES _____

I have exercised...

DOING?	TIME	Calories Burned

TOTAL CALORIES BURNED _____

I have slept...

_____ HOURS

I have drank...

CUPS OF WATER

Meds/vitamins taken

FINAL CALORIES _____
(Calories eaten - calories burned)

Weight today? _____

Change? +/- _____

Date _____

How are you feeling today? _____

I have eaten...			I have exercised...		
BREAKFAST	WHAT TIME?	Calories	DOING?	TIME	Calories Burned
LUNCH	WHAT TIME?	Calories			

TOTAL CALORIES BURNED _____

I have slept...

DINNER	WHAT TIME?	Calories

_____ HOURS

I have drank...

_____ CUPS OF WATER

Meds/vitamins taken

SNACKS	WHAT TIME?	Calories

TOTAL CALORIES _____   **FINAL CALORIES** _____
(Calories eaten - calories burned)

Weight today? _____   **Change? +/-** _____

Date _____

How are you feeling today? _____

I have eaten...

BREAKFAST	WHAT TIME?	Calories

LUNCH	WHAT TIME?	Calories

DINNER	WHAT TIME?	Calories

SNACKS	WHAT TIME?	Calories

TOTAL CALORIES _____

I have exercised...

DOING?	TIME	Calories Burned

TOTAL CALORIES BURNED _____

I have slept...

_____ HOURS

I have drank...

_____ CUPS OF WATER

Meds/vitamins taken

_____

_____

_____

FINAL CALORIES _____
(Calories eaten - calories burned)

Weight today? _____   ## Change? +/- _____

Date _____

How are you feeling today? _____

I have eaten...

BREAKFAST	WHAT TIME?	Calories

LUNCH	WHAT TIME?	Calories

DINNER	WHAT TIME?	Calories

SNACKS	WHAT TIME?	Calories

TOTAL CALORIES _____

I have exercised...

DOING?	TIME	Calories Burned

TOTAL CALORIES BURNED _____

I have slept...

_____ HOURS

I have drank...

_____ CUPS OF WATER

Meds/vitamins taken

_____

_____

_____

FINAL CALORIES _____
(Calories eaten - calories burned)

Weight today? _____ # Change? +/- _____

Date _____

How are you feeling today? _____

I have eaten...

BREAKFAST	WHAT TIME?	Calories

LUNCH	WHAT TIME?	Calories

DINNER	WHAT TIME?	Calories

SNACKS	WHAT TIME?	Calories

TOTAL CALORIES _____

I have exercised...

DOING?	TIME	Calories Burned

TOTAL CALORIES BURNED _____

I have slept...

_____ HOURS

I have drank...

_____ CUPS OF WATER

Meds/vitamins taken

_____

_____

_____

_____

FINAL CALORIES _____
(Calories eaten - calories burned)

Weight today? _____ ## Change? +/- _____

Date _____

How are you feeling today? _____

I have eaten...

BREAKFAST	WHAT TIME?	Calories

LUNCH	WHAT TIME?	Calories

DINNER	WHAT TIME?	Calories

SNACKS	WHAT TIME?	Calories

TOTAL CALORIES _____

I have exercised...

DOING?	TIME	Calories Burned

TOTAL CALORIES BURNED _____

I have slept...

_____ HOURS

I have drank...

_____ CUPS OF WATER

Meds/vitamins taken

FINAL CALORIES _____
(Calories eaten - calories burned)

Weight today? _____   # Change? +/- _____

Date _____

How are you feeling today? _____

I have eaten...

BREAKFAST	WHAT TIME?	Calories

LUNCH	WHAT TIME?	Calories

DINNER	WHAT TIME?	Calories

SNACKS	WHAT TIME?	Calories

TOTAL CALORIES _____

I have exercised...

DOING?	TIME	Calories Burned

TOTAL CALORIES BURNED _____

I have slept...

_____ HOURS

I have drank...

CUPS OF WATER

Meds/vitamins taken

FINAL CALORIES _____
(Calories eaten - calories burned)

Weight today? _____   ## Change? +/- _____

Date _____

How are you feeling today? _____

I have eaten...

BREAKFAST	WHAT TIME?	Calories

LUNCH	WHAT TIME?	Calories

DINNER	WHAT TIME?	Calories

SNACKS	WHAT TIME?	Calories

TOTAL CALORIES _____

I have exercised...

DOING?	TIME	Calories Burned

TOTAL CALORIES BURNED _____

I have slept...

_____ HOURS

I have drank...

_____ CUPS OF WATER

Meds/vitamins taken

FINAL CALORIES _____
(Calories eaten - calories burned)

Weight today? _____   Change? +/- _____

Date _____

How are you feeling today? _____

I have eaten...

BREAKFAST	WHAT TIME?	Calories

LUNCH	WHAT TIME?	Calories

DINNER	WHAT TIME?	Calories

SNACKS	WHAT TIME?	Calories

TOTAL CALORIES _____

I have exercised...

DOING?	TIME	Calories Burned

TOTAL CALORIES BURNED _____

I have slept...

_____ HOURS

I have drank...

CUPS OF WATER

Meds/vitamins taken

FINAL CALORIES _____
(Calories eaten - calories burned)

Weight today? _____

Change? +/- _____

Date _____

How are you feeling today? _____

I have eaten...

BREAKFAST	WHAT TIME?	Calories

LUNCH	WHAT TIME?	Calories

DINNER	WHAT TIME?	Calories

SNACKS	WHAT TIME?	Calories

TOTAL CALORIES _____

I have exercised...

DOING?	TIME	Calories Burned

TOTAL CALORIES BURNED _____

I have slept...

HOURS _____

I have drank...

CUPS OF WATER _____

Meds/vitamins taken

_____

_____

_____

FINAL CALORIES _____
(Calories eaten - calories burned)

Weight today? _____   ## Change? +/- _____

Date _____

How are you feeling today? _____

I have eaten...

BREAKFAST	WHAT TIME?	Calories

LUNCH	WHAT TIME?	Calories

DINNER	WHAT TIME?	Calories

SNACKS	WHAT TIME?	Calories

TOTAL CALORIES _____

I have exercised...

DOING?	TIME	Calories Burned

TOTAL CALORIES BURNED _____

I have slept...

_____ HOURS

I have drank...

CUPS OF WATER

Meds/vitamins taken

_____
_____
_____

FINAL CALORIES _____
(Calories eaten - calories burned)

Weight today? _____   **Change? +/-** _____

Date _____

How are you feeling today? _____

I have eaten...

BREAKFAST	WHAT TIME?	Calories

LUNCH	WHAT TIME?	Calories

DINNER	WHAT TIME?	Calories

SNACKS	WHAT TIME?	Calories

TOTAL CALORIES _____

Weight today? _____

I have exercised...

DOING?	TIME	Calories Burned

TOTAL CALORIES BURNED _____

I have slept...

_____ HOURS

I have drank...

_____ CUPS OF WATER

Meds/vitamins taken

_____
_____
_____
_____

FINAL CALORIES _____
(Calories eaten - calories burned)

Change? +/- _____

Date _____

How are you feeling today? _____

I have eaten...

BREAKFAST	WHAT TIME?	Calories

LUNCH	WHAT TIME?	Calories

DINNER	WHAT TIME?	Calories

SNACKS	WHAT TIME?	Calories

TOTAL CALORIES _____

I have exercised...

DOING?	TIME	Calories Burned

TOTAL CALORIES BURNED _____

I have slept...
_____ HOURS

I have drank...
_____ CUPS OF WATER

Meds/vitamins taken
_____
_____
_____
_____

FINAL CALORIES _____
(Calories eaten - calories burned)

Weight today? _____ **Change? +/-** _____

Date

How are you feeling today?

I have eaten...

BREAKFAST	WHAT TIME?	Calories

LUNCH	WHAT TIME?	Calories

DINNER	WHAT TIME?	Calories

SNACKS	WHAT TIME?	Calories

TOTAL CALORIES

Weight today?

I have exercised...

DOING?	TIME	Calories Burned

TOTAL CALORIES BURNED

I have slept...

HOURS

I have drank...

CUPS OF WATER

Meds/vitamins taken

FINAL CALORIES
(Calories eaten - calories burned)

Change? +/-

Date _____

How are you feeling today? _____

I have eaten...			I have exercised...		
BREAKFAST	WHAT TIME?	Calories	DOING?	TIME	Calories Burned
LUNCH	WHAT TIME?	Calories			
			TOTAL CALORIES BURNED _____		
			I have slept...		
DINNER	WHAT TIME?	Calories			HOURS
			I have drank...		
					CUPS OF WATER
			Meds/vitamins taken		
SNACKS	WHAT TIME?	Calories			

TOTAL CALORIES _____

FINAL CALORIES _____
(Calories eaten - calories burned)

Weight today? _____   **Change? +/-** _____

Date _____

How are you feeling today? _____

I have eaten...

BREAKFAST	WHAT TIME?	Calories

LUNCH	WHAT TIME?	Calories

DINNER	WHAT TIME?	Calories

SNACKS	WHAT TIME?	Calories

TOTAL CALORIES _____

I have exercised...

DOING?	TIME	Calories Burned

TOTAL CALORIES BURNED _____

I have slept...

_____ HOURS

I have drank...

_____ CUPS OF WATER

Meds/vitamins taken

_____

_____

_____

FINAL CALORIES _____
(Calories eaten - calories burned)

Weight today? _____   ## Change? +/- _____

Date _____

How are you feeling today? _____

I have eaten...

BREAKFAST	WHAT TIME?	Calories

LUNCH	WHAT TIME?	Calories

DINNER	WHAT TIME?	Calories

SNACKS	WHAT TIME?	Calories

TOTAL CALORIES _____

Weight today? _____

I have exercised...

DOING?	TIME	Calories Burned

TOTAL CALORIES BURNED _____

I have slept...

_____ HOURS

I have drank...

_____ CUPS OF WATER

Meds/vitamins taken

_____

_____

_____

FINAL CALORIES _____
(Calories eaten - calories burned)

Change? +/- _____

Date _____

How are you feeling today? _____

I have eaten...

BREAKFAST	WHAT TIME?	Calories

LUNCH	WHAT TIME?	Calories

DINNER	WHAT TIME?	Calories

SNACKS	WHAT TIME?	Calories

TOTAL CALORIES _____

I have exercised...

DOING?	TIME	Calories Burned

TOTAL CALORIES BURNED _____

I have slept...

_____ **HOURS**

I have drank...

_____ **CUPS OF WATER**

Meds/vitamins taken

_____

_____

_____

FINAL CALORIES _____
(Calories eaten - calories burned)

Weight today? _____   ## Change? +/- _____

Date _____

How are you feeling today? _____

I have eaten...		
BREAKFAST	WHAT TIME?	Calories
LUNCH	WHAT TIME?	Calories
DINNER	WHAT TIME?	Calories
SNACKS	WHAT TIME?	Calories

TOTAL CALORIES _____

Weight today? _____

I have exercised...		
DOING?	TIME	Calories Burned

TOTAL CALORIES BURNED _____

I have slept...

HOURS _____

I have drank...

CUPS OF WATER

Meds/vitamins taken

FINAL CALORIES _____
(Calories eaten - calories burned)

Change? +/- _____

Date _____

How are you feeling today? _____

I have eaten...

BREAKFAST	WHAT TIME?	Calories
LUNCH	WHAT TIME?	Calories
DINNER	WHAT TIME?	Calories
SNACKS	WHAT TIME?	Calories

TOTAL CALORIES

I have exercised...

DOING?	TIME	Calories Burned

TOTAL CALORIES BURNED _____

I have slept...

HOURS _____

I have drank...

CUPS OF WATER _____

Meds/vitamins taken

_____
_____
_____
_____

FINAL CALORIES
(Calories eaten - calories burned)

Weight today? _____   **Change? +/-** _____

Date _____

How are you feeling today? _____

I have eaten...

BREAKFAST	WHAT TIME?	Calories

LUNCH	WHAT TIME?	Calories

DINNER	WHAT TIME?	Calories

SNACKS	WHAT TIME?	Calories

TOTAL CALORIES _____

I have exercised...

DOING?	TIME	Calories Burned

TOTAL CALORIES BURNED _____

I have slept...

_____ HOURS

I have drank...

_____ CUPS OF WATER

Meds/vitamins taken

_____

FINAL CALORIES _____
(Calories eaten - calories burned)

Weight today? _____

Change? +/- _____

Date _____

How are you feeling today? _____

I have eaten...

BREAKFAST	WHAT TIME?	Calories

LUNCH	WHAT TIME?	Calories

DINNER	WHAT TIME?	Calories

SNACKS	WHAT TIME?	Calories

TOTAL CALORIES

I have exercised...

DOING?	TIME	Calories Burned

TOTAL CALORIES BURNED _____

I have slept...

_____ HOURS

I have drank...

CUPS OF WATER

Meds/vitamins taken

FINAL CALORIES
(Calories eaten - calories burned)

Weight today? _____

Change? +/- _____

Date _____

How are you feeling today? _____

I have eaten...		
BREAKFAST	**WHAT TIME?**	Calories
LUNCH	**WHAT TIME?**	Calories
DINNER	**WHAT TIME?**	Calories
SNACKS	**WHAT TIME?**	Calories
TOTAL CALORIES	_____	

I have exercised...

DOING?	**TIME**	Calories Burned

TOTAL CALORIES BURNED _____

I have slept...

_____ HOURS

I have drank...

CUPS OF WATER

Meds/vitamins taken

FINAL CALORIES _____
(Calories eaten - calories burned)

Weight today? _____   ## Change? +/- _____

Date _____

How are you feeling today? _____

I have eaten...

BREAKFAST	WHAT TIME?	Calories

LUNCH	WHAT TIME?	Calories

DINNER	WHAT TIME?	Calories

SNACKS	WHAT TIME?	Calories

TOTAL CALORIES _____

I have exercised...

DOING?	TIME	Calories Burned

TOTAL CALORIES BURNED _____

I have slept...

_____ HOURS

I have drank...

_____ CUPS OF WATER

Meds/vitamins taken

_____
_____
_____
_____

FINAL CALORIES _____
(Calories eaten - calories burned)

Weight today? _____   # Change? +/- _____

Date _____

How are you feeling today? _____

I have eaten...

BREAKFAST	WHAT TIME?	Calories

LUNCH	WHAT TIME?	Calories

DINNER	WHAT TIME?	Calories

SNACKS	WHAT TIME?	Calories

TOTAL CALORIES _____

I have exercised...

DOING?	TIME	Calories Burned

TOTAL CALORIES BURNED _____

I have slept...

_____ **HOURS**

I have drank...

_____ **CUPS OF WATER**

Meds/vitamins taken

_____

_____

_____

FINAL CALORIES _____
(Calories eaten - calories burned)

Weight today? _____

Change? +/- _____

Date _____

How are you feeling today? _____

I have eaten...				I have exercised...		
BREAKFAST	WHAT TIME?	Calories		DOING?	TIME	Calories Burned
LUNCH	WHAT TIME?	Calories				
				TOTAL CALORIES BURNED _____		

I have slept...

DINNER   WHAT TIME?   Calories   HOURS _____

I have drank...

CUPS OF WATER _____

Meds/vitamins taken

SNACKS   WHAT TIME?   Calories

TOTAL CALORIES _____   **FINAL CALORIES** _____
(Calories eaten - calories burned)

Weight today? _____   **Change? +/-** _____

Date

How are you feeling today?

I have eaten...

BREAKFAST	WHAT TIME?	Calories

LUNCH	WHAT TIME?	Calories

DINNER	WHAT TIME?	Calories

SNACKS	WHAT TIME?	Calories

TOTAL CALORIES

Weight today?

I have exercised...

DOING?	TIME	Calories Burned

TOTAL CALORIES BURNED

I have slept...

HOURS

I have drank...

CUPS OF WATER

Meds/vitamins taken

FINAL CALORIES
(Calories eaten - calories burned)

Change? +/-

Date

How are you feeling today?

I have eaten...

BREAKFAST	WHAT TIME?	Calories

LUNCH	WHAT TIME?	Calories

DINNER	WHAT TIME?	Calories

SNACKS	WHAT TIME?	Calories

TOTAL CALORIES

I have exercised...

DOING?	TIME	Calories Burned

TOTAL CALORIES BURNED

I have slept...

HOURS

I have drank...

CUPS OF WATER

Meds/vitamins taken

FINAL CALORIES
(Calories eaten - calories burned)

Weight today?   **Change? +/-**

Date _____

How are you feeling today? _____

I have eaten...

BREAKFAST	WHAT TIME?	Calories

LUNCH	WHAT TIME?	Calories

DINNER	WHAT TIME?	Calories

SNACKS	WHAT TIME?	Calories

TOTAL CALORIES _____

I have exercised...

DOING?	TIME	Calories Burned

TOTAL CALORIES BURNED _____

I have slept...

_____ HOURS

I have drank...

_____ CUPS OF WATER

Meds/vitamins taken

_____
_____
_____
_____

FINAL CALORIES _____
(Calories eaten - calories burned)

Weight today? _____

Change? +/- _____

Date _____

How are you feeling today? _____

I have eaten...

BREAKFAST	WHAT TIME?	Calories

LUNCH	WHAT TIME?	Calories

DINNER	WHAT TIME?	Calories

SNACKS	WHAT TIME?	Calories

TOTAL CALORIES

I have exercised...

DOING?	TIME	Calories Burned

TOTAL CALORIES BURNED _____

I have slept...

_____ HOURS

I have drank...

CUPS OF WATER

Meds/vitamins taken

_____

_____

_____

FINAL CALORIES _____
(Calories eaten - calories burned)

Weight today? _____   ## Change? +/- _____

Date _____

How are you feeling today? _____

I have eaten...

BREAKFAST	WHAT TIME?	Calories

LUNCH	WHAT TIME?	Calories

DINNER	WHAT TIME?	Calories

SNACKS	WHAT TIME?	Calories

TOTAL CALORIES _____

I have exercised...

DOING?	TIME	Calories Burned

TOTAL CALORIES BURNED _____

I have slept...

_____ HOURS

I have drank...

_____ CUPS OF WATER

Meds/vitamins taken

_____

_____

_____

_____

FINAL CALORIES _____
(Calories eaten - calories burned)

Weight today? _____

Change? +/- _____

Date _____

How are you feeling today? _____

I have eaten...

BREAKFAST	WHAT TIME?	Calories
LUNCH	WHAT TIME?	Calories
DINNER	WHAT TIME?	Calories
SNACKS	WHAT TIME?	Calories

TOTAL CALORIES

Weight today? _____

I have exercised...

DOING?	TIME	Calories Burned

TOTAL CALORIES BURNED _____

I have slept...

_____ **HOURS**

I have drank...

_____ **CUPS OF WATER**

Meds/vitamins taken

_____

_____

_____

_____

FINAL CALORIES _____
(Calories eaten - calories burned)

Change? +/- _____

Date _____

How are you feeling today? _____

I have eaten...

BREAKFAST	WHAT TIME?	Calories

LUNCH	WHAT TIME?	Calories

DINNER	WHAT TIME?	Calories

SNACKS	WHAT TIME?	Calories

TOTAL CALORIES _____

I have exercised...

DOING?	TIME	Calories Burned

TOTAL CALORIES BURNED _____

I have slept...

_____ HOURS

I have drank...

_____ CUPS OF WATER

Meds/vitamins taken

_____

_____

_____

FINAL CALORIES _____
(Calories eaten - calories burned)

Weight today? _____

Change? +/- _____

Date _____

How are you feeling today? _____

I have eaten...

BREAKFAST	WHAT TIME?	Calories

LUNCH	WHAT TIME?	Calories

DINNER	WHAT TIME?	Calories

SNACKS	WHAT TIME?	Calories

TOTAL CALORIES _____

I have exercised...

DOING?	TIME	Calories Burned

TOTAL CALORIES BURNED _____

I have slept...

_____ HOURS

I have drank...

_____ CUPS OF WATER

Meds/vitamins taken

_____

_____

_____

FINAL CALORIES _____
(Calories eaten - calories burned)

Weight today? _____

Change? +/- _____

Date _____

How are you feeling today? _____

I have eaten...

BREAKFAST	WHAT TIME?	Calories

LUNCH	WHAT TIME?	Calories

DINNER	WHAT TIME?	Calories

SNACKS	WHAT TIME?	Calories

TOTAL CALORIES _____

I have exercised...

DOING?	TIME	Calories Burned

TOTAL CALORIES BURNED _____

I have slept...

_____ HOURS

I have drank...

_____ CUPS OF WATER

Meds/vitamins taken

_____
_____
_____
_____

FINAL CALORIES _____
(Calories eaten - calories burned)

Weight today? _____   ## Change? +/- _____

Date _____

How are you feeling today? _____

I have eaten...

BREAKFAST	WHAT TIME?	Calories

LUNCH	WHAT TIME?	Calories

DINNER	WHAT TIME?	Calories

SNACKS	WHAT TIME?	Calories

TOTAL CALORIES _____

I have exercised...

DOING?	TIME	Calories Burned

TOTAL CALORIES BURNED _____

I have slept...

_____ HOURS

I have drank...

_____ CUPS OF WATER

Meds/vitamins taken

_____

FINAL CALORIES _____
(Calories eaten - calories burned)

Weight today? _____

Change? +/- _____

Date _____

How are you feeling today? _____

I have eaten...

BREAKFAST	WHAT TIME?	Calories

LUNCH	WHAT TIME?	Calories

DINNER	WHAT TIME?	Calories

SNACKS	WHAT TIME?	Calories

TOTAL CALORIES _____

I have exercised...

DOING?	TIME	Calories Burned

TOTAL CALORIES BURNED _____

I have slept...

_____ HOURS

I have drank...

_____ CUPS OF WATER

Meds/vitamins taken

_____

_____

_____

FINAL CALORIES _____
(Calories eaten - calories burned)

Weight today? _____

Change? +/- _____

Date _____

How are you feeling today? _____

I have eaten...

BREAKFAST	WHAT TIME?	Calories

LUNCH	WHAT TIME?	Calories

DINNER	WHAT TIME?	Calories

SNACKS	WHAT TIME?	Calories

TOTAL CALORIES _____

I have exercised...

DOING?	TIME	Calories Burned

TOTAL CALORIES BURNED _____

I have slept...

_____ HOURS

I have drank...

_____ CUPS OF WATER

Meds/vitamins taken

_____

_____

_____

FINAL CALORIES _____
(Calories eaten - calories burned)

Weight today? _____   **Change? +/-** _____

Date _____

How are you feeling today? _____

I have eaten...

BREAKFAST	WHAT TIME?	Calories

LUNCH	WHAT TIME?	Calories

DINNER	WHAT TIME?	Calories

SNACKS	WHAT TIME?	Calories

TOTAL CALORIES _____

Weight today? _____

I have exercised...

DOING?	TIME	Calories Burned

TOTAL CALORIES BURNED _____

I have slept...

_____ **HOURS**

I have drank...

_____ **CUPS OF WATER**

Meds/vitamins taken

_____

_____

_____

_____

FINAL CALORIES _____
(Calories eaten - calories burned)

Change? +/- _____

Date _____

How are you feeling today? _____

I have eaten...   ## I have exercised...

BREAKFAST	WHAT TIME?	Calories		DOING?	TIME	Calories Burned

LUNCH   **WHAT TIME?**   Calories

TOTAL CALORIES BURNED _____

I have slept...

DINNER   **WHAT TIME?**   Calories

HOURS _____

I have drank...

CUPS OF WATER _____

Meds/vitamins taken

SNACKS   **WHAT TIME?**   Calories

TOTAL CALORIES _____   **FINAL CALORIES** _____

(Calories eaten - calories burned)

Weight today? _____   ## Change? +/- _____

Date _____

How are you feeling today? _____

I have eaten...

BREAKFAST	WHAT TIME?	Calories

LUNCH	WHAT TIME?	Calories

DINNER	WHAT TIME?	Calories

SNACKS	WHAT TIME?	Calories

TOTAL CALORIES _____

Weight today? _____

I have exercised...

DOING?	TIME	Calories Burned

TOTAL CALORIES BURNED _____

I have slept...

_____ HOURS

I have drank...

_____ CUPS OF WATER

Meds/vitamins taken

_____

_____

_____

FINAL CALORIES _____
(Calories eaten - calories burned)

Change? +/- _____

Date _____

How are you feeling today? _____

I have eaten...

BREAKFAST	WHAT TIME?	Calories

LUNCH	WHAT TIME?	Calories

DINNER	WHAT TIME?	Calories

SNACKS	WHAT TIME?	Calories

TOTAL CALORIES _____

I have exercised...

DOING?	TIME	Calories Burned

TOTAL CALORIES BURNED _____

I have slept...

_____ HOURS

I have drank...

_____ CUPS OF WATER

Meds/vitamins taken

_____

_____

_____

FINAL CALORIES _____
(Calories eaten - calories burned)

Weight today? _____   ## Change? +/- _____

Date _____

How are you feeling today? _____

I have eaten...			I have exercised...		
BREAKFAST	**WHAT TIME?**	Calories	DOING?	**TIME**	Calories Burned
LUNCH	**WHAT TIME?**	Calories			
			TOTAL CALORIES BURNED _____		

I have slept...

_____ **HOURS**

DINNER	**WHAT TIME?**	Calories

I have drank...

CUPS OF WATER

Meds/vitamins taken

SNACKS	**WHAT TIME?**	Calories

TOTAL CALORIES _____

FINAL CALORIES _____
(Calories eaten - calories burned)

Weight today? _____   **Change? +/-** _____

Date _____

How are you feeling today? _____

I have eaten...   # I have exercised...

BREAKFAST	WHAT TIME?	Calories

LUNCH	WHAT TIME?	Calories

DINNER	WHAT TIME?	Calories

SNACKS	WHAT TIME?	Calories

TOTAL CALORIES

DOING?	TIME	Calories Burned

TOTAL CALORIES BURNED _____

I have slept...

_____ HOURS

I have drank...

_____ CUPS OF WATER

Meds/vitamins taken

_____
_____
_____
_____

FINAL CALORIES _____
(Calories eaten - calories burned)

Weight today? _____   # Change? +/- _____

Date _____

How are you feeling today? _____

I have eaten...

BREAKFAST	WHAT TIME?	Calories

LUNCH	WHAT TIME?	Calories

DINNER	WHAT TIME?	Calories

SNACKS	WHAT TIME?	Calories

TOTAL CALORIES _____

I have exercised...

DOING?	TIME	Calories Burned

TOTAL CALORIES BURNED _____

I have slept...

_____ HOURS

I have drank...

_____ CUPS OF WATER

Meds/vitamins taken

_____

FINAL CALORIES _____
(Calories eaten - calories burned)

Weight today? _____

Change? +/- _____

Date _____

How are you feeling today? _____

I have eaten...

BREAKFAST	WHAT TIME?	Calories

LUNCH	WHAT TIME?	Calories

DINNER	WHAT TIME?	Calories

SNACKS	WHAT TIME?	Calories

TOTAL CALORIES

I have exercised...

DOING?	TIME	Calories Burned

TOTAL CALORIES BURNED _____

I have slept...

_____ HOURS

I have drank...

_____ CUPS OF WATER

Meds/vitamins taken

FINAL CALORIES _____
(Calories eaten - calories burned)

Weight today? _____

Change? +/- _____

Date _____

How are you feeling today? _____

I have eaten...

BREAKFAST	WHAT TIME?	Calories

LUNCH	WHAT TIME?	Calories

DINNER	WHAT TIME?	Calories

SNACKS	WHAT TIME?	Calories

TOTAL CALORIES _____

Weight today? _____

I have exercised...

DOING?	TIME	Calories Burned

TOTAL CALORIES BURNED _____

I have slept...

_____ HOURS

I have drank...

_____ CUPS OF WATER

Meds/vitamins taken

_____

_____

FINAL CALORIES _____
(Calories eaten - calories burned)

Change? +/- _____

Date _____

How are you feeling today? _____

I have eaten...

BREAKFAST	WHAT TIME?	Calories

LUNCH	WHAT TIME?	Calories

DINNER	WHAT TIME?	Calories

SNACKS	WHAT TIME?	Calories

TOTAL CALORIES _____

I have exercised...

DOING?	TIME	Calories Burned

TOTAL CALORIES BURNED _____

I have slept...

_____ HOURS

I have drank...

_____ CUPS OF WATER

Meds/vitamins taken

_____
_____
_____
_____

FINAL CALORIES _____
(Calories eaten - calories burned)

Weight today? _____   ## Change? +/- _____

Date _____

How are you feeling today? _____

I have eaten...			I have exercised...		
BREAKFAST	WHAT TIME?	Calories	DOING?	TIME	Calories Burned
LUNCH	WHAT TIME?	Calories			
			TOTAL CALORIES BURNED _____		
			I have slept...		
DINNER	WHAT TIME?	Calories			HOURS
			_____		
			I have drank...		
					CUPS OF WATER
			Meds/vitamins taken		
SNACKS	WHAT TIME?	Calories			
TOTAL CALORIES _____			**FINAL CALORIES** _____ (Calories eaten - calories burned)		

Weight today? _____   **Change? +/-** _____

Date _____

How are you feeling today? _____

I have eaten...

BREAKFAST	WHAT TIME?	Calories

LUNCH	WHAT TIME?	Calories

DINNER	WHAT TIME?	Calories

SNACKS	WHAT TIME?	Calories

TOTAL CALORIES _____

I have exercised...

DOING?	TIME	Calories Burned

TOTAL CALORIES BURNED _____

I have slept...

_____ HOURS

I have drank...

_____ CUPS OF WATER

Meds/vitamins taken

_____
_____
_____
_____

FINAL CALORIES _____
(Calories eaten - calories burned)

Weight today? _____   # Change? +/- _____

Date _____

How are you feeling today? _____

I have eaten...

BREAKFAST	WHAT TIME?	Calories

LUNCH	WHAT TIME?	Calories

DINNER	WHAT TIME?	Calories

SNACKS	WHAT TIME?	Calories

TOTAL CALORIES _____

I have exercised...

DOING?	TIME	Calories Burned

TOTAL CALORIES BURNED _____

I have slept...

_____ HOURS

I have drank...

_____ CUPS OF WATER

Meds/vitamins taken

_____

_____

_____

FINAL CALORIES _____
(Calories eaten - calories burned)

Weight today? _____

Change? +/- _____

Date _____

How are you feeling today? _____

I have eaten...

BREAKFAST	WHAT TIME?	Calories

LUNCH	WHAT TIME?	Calories

DINNER	WHAT TIME?	Calories

SNACKS	WHAT TIME?	Calories

TOTAL CALORIES _____

I have exercised...

DOING?	TIME	Calories Burned

TOTAL CALORIES BURNED _____

I have slept...

_____ HOURS

I have drank...

_____ CUPS OF WATER

Meds/vitamins taken

_____

_____

_____

_____

FINAL CALORIES _____
(Calories eaten - calories burned)

Weight today? _____

Change? +/- _____

Date _____

How are you feeling today? _____

I have eaten...   # I have exercised...

BREAKFAST	WHAT TIME?	Calories	DOING?	TIME	Calories Burned

LUNCH	WHAT TIME?	Calories

TOTAL CALORIES BURNED _____

I have slept...

_____ **HOURS**

DINNER	WHAT TIME?	Calories

I have drank...

_____ **CUPS OF WATER**

Meds/vitamins taken

SNACKS	WHAT TIME?	Calories

TOTAL CALORIES _____

FINAL CALORIES _____
(Calories eaten - calories burned)

Weight today? _____   **Change? +/-** _____

Date _____

How are you feeling today? _____

I have eaten...

BREAKFAST	WHAT TIME?	Calories

LUNCH	WHAT TIME?	Calories

DINNER	WHAT TIME?	Calories

SNACKS	WHAT TIME?	Calories

TOTAL CALORIES

I have exercised...

DOING?	TIME	Calories Burned

TOTAL CALORIES BURNED _____

I have slept...

HOURS _____

I have drank...

CUPS OF WATER _____

Meds/vitamins taken

FINAL CALORIES
(Calories eaten - calories burned)

Weight today? _____   **Change? +/-** _____

Date _____

How are you feeling today? _____

I have eaten...

BREAKFAST	WHAT TIME?	Calories

LUNCH	WHAT TIME?	Calories

DINNER	WHAT TIME?	Calories

SNACKS	WHAT TIME?	Calories

TOTAL CALORIES _____

I have exercised...

DOING?	TIME	Calories Burned

TOTAL CALORIES BURNED _____

I have slept...

_____ HOURS

I have drank...

_____ CUPS OF WATER

Meds/vitamins taken

FINAL CALORIES _____
(Calories eaten - calories burned)

Weight today? _____

Change? +/- _____

Date _____

How are you feeling today? _____

I have eaten...

BREAKFAST	WHAT TIME?	Calories

LUNCH	WHAT TIME?	Calories

DINNER	WHAT TIME?	Calories

SNACKS	WHAT TIME?	Calories

TOTAL CALORIES _____

Weight today? _____

I have exercised...

DOING?	TIME	Calories Burned

TOTAL CALORIES BURNED _____

I have slept...

_____ HOURS

I have drank...

_____ CUPS OF WATER

Meds/vitamins taken

_____

_____

_____

FINAL CALORIES _____
(Calories eaten - calories burned)

Change? +/- _____

Date _____

How are you feeling today? _____

I have eaten...

BREAKFAST	WHAT TIME?	Calories

LUNCH	WHAT TIME?	Calories

DINNER	WHAT TIME?	Calories

SNACKS	WHAT TIME?	Calories

TOTAL CALORIES _____

I have exercised...

DOING?	TIME	Calories Burned

TOTAL CALORIES BURNED _____

I have slept...

_____ HOURS

I have drank...

_____ CUPS OF WATER

Meds/vitamins taken

FINAL CALORIES _____
(Calories eaten - calories burned)

Weight today? _____

Change? +/- _____

Date _____

How are you feeling today? _____

I have eaten...

BREAKFAST	WHAT TIME?	Calories

LUNCH	WHAT TIME?	Calories

DINNER	WHAT TIME?	Calories

SNACKS	WHAT TIME?	Calories

TOTAL CALORIES _____

I have exercised...

DOING?	TIME	Calories Burned

TOTAL CALORIES BURNED _____

I have slept...

_____ HOURS

I have drank...

_____ CUPS OF WATER

Meds/vitamins taken

_____

_____

_____

FINAL CALORIES _____
(Calories eaten - calories burned)

Weight today? _____   **Change? +/-** _____

46360510R00051

Printed in Poland
by Amazon Fulfillment
Poland Sp. z o.o., Wrocław